HYPERTENSION? BLOOD SUGAR? DEPRESSION? HOW I CURED THEM ALL

My Personal Story

Leonid Altshuler M.D.

Important Notice

The **information** in this book is not intended or implied to be a substitute for professional medical **advice**, **diagnosis** or **treatment**. All content, including text, graphics, images and **information**, available in this book is for general **information** purposes only.

NEVER STOP TAKING YOUR MEDICATIONS WITHOUT CONSULTING WITH YOUR DOCTOR

AUTHOR'S NOTE

This is not a book of facts and figures, or graphs and charts. This is my opinion based on my own personal experience, and after many years seeing patients in my profession as a psychiatrist. I do not use complicated terms, or scientific jargon. This is a simple book so readers can understand the concept and implement the changes I recommend. Of course, further reading can and should be done on the topic, but with this book you can get started on changing your life for the better.

CONTENTS

INTRODUCTION

A well-known and well-researched illness effectively kills millions of people all over the world. The illness starts slowly. It initially presents with different symptoms that have a tendency to significantly worsen over an extremely long period. It usually takes several years for the physical symptoms to appear and for laboratory tests results to become evident, and eventually for doctors to make a definite diagnosis. Patients are generally treated according to the symptoms they experience. This is what happened to me. My doctors were good. They did everything they could. They could not do more because the real cause of my problems remained a mystery. Finally, it was concluded that my symptoms were psychosomatic — caused by stress.

In this book, I want to share my story with readers. My experience is not unique. Millions of people probably share this same story.

This book may not have enough pages to be properly called a book. This is done intentionally because I have given value to each word. This means that I say only what is necessary for the reader to know, and nothing else. Why is this important? It is vital, because in general people are drawn into oceans of information that can be confusing. Very quickly, they do not know what to believe and to whom they should listen. I am not saying that people need to listen to what I write. Absolutely not. My point is that when it comes to health, people need to be able to focus their attention on the most important things. People need to be able to find the source and the cause of their health problems. They need to consult doctors and other medical specialists to find out what is wrong with them, but they also need knowledge. My purpose here is to direct the reader's attention to the most important details so they know what issues to bring up and discuss with their primary care providers.

This book is short because I am not going to write thousands of pages, copying information that can be readily obtained on websites and anywhere else.

Again, I will be directing the attention of the reader to specific websites on the Internet: websites I consider important from an educational point of view. I will provide links to those places on my own website, so readers can remain focused.

Leonid Altshuler M.D.

CHAPTER 1

Who is Leonid Altshuler, MD?

You may wonder who I am. I am a Board Certified Psychiatrist who has been practicing for over twenty-five years. During this time, I have seen thousands of patients with different mental health issues. I gained experience in the treatment of illnesses, using different types of medication, and psychotherapy. Just as importantly, I have been educating myself about the latest research conducted in my area of expertise. What I have learned and discovered in the area of brain research is so important that I want to share it with others. This will give readers some critical information and pointers they can discuss when visiting their primary care provider.

Why did I decide to write this book?

I decided to write this book to share my knowledge and personal experience. After many years of suffering from several health issues, I discovered

4

the cause through my own research and I recovered completely within less than one month. This recovery included both my mental and physical wellbeing. It was an experiment I performed on myself that turned out to be extremely successful. Please note that I do not recommend anyone attempt such an experiment on himself or herself or anyone else, without first talking to his or her primary health provider.

I want to educate the reader about the main reason why I suffered for so many years. I want to discuss the main reason the doctors who were treating me did not give me the right diagnosis. I also want to address the main reason I was not able to find the diagnosis myself. How did this happen in spite of the fact that so many well trained doctors saw me? How could this happen?

Why did it happen, when the reason I was having all those symptoms and problems was not only obvious, but had been well-known for a long time and even studied in detail.

I did not have the answers to these questions. It took me a long time, through meditation and research, to find the answers.

The main reason I want to write this book is to direct the reader's attention to one of the main and most important causes of all health problems in this modern society in which we live. My book is purely educational and designed to help people to acquire knowledge that allows them to stay healthy and happy.

Why my growing up in Russia is important to mention

Growing up in Russia was not simple. Most of the time you must rely on yourself for everything you do. For example, when something breaks down at home, it is almost impossible to get someone to repair it. This means you need to learn about all sorts of things, and at times you even need to become some type of plumber or electrician or any other type of specialized worker. If you want to have nice clothes you need to be inventive and use all of your intelligence to be able to figure out how and where to get clothes you could wear without feeling ashamed. The same applies to getting food, and I could go on, and on, and on... The bottom line is that most of the time growing up, I needed to rely on myself to come up with a solution to a problem. Luckily for me, I retained that useful habit throughout my life, and this is what helped me find the answer to my on-going health issues.

At some point in my life, after years of traveling from one doctor's office to another, I finally gave up this adventure and decided I needed to use my self-reliance skills only, and not rely on anything or anybody else.

Why did it take me so long? I have a hard time answering this question, but I suspect I was not really thinking much, because I was always busy, running around trying to accomplish many tasks at the same time, being distracted by a thousand things, not being able to calm down and focus my attention on the most important issue in my life.

CHAPTER 2

The beginning: My health issues

I was always scared of being sick. My father became extremely ill when I was a small child growing up back in the USSR. I was exposed to his suffering and it had a great impact on me emotionally. As a result, I did everything possible to stay healthy myself. I paid attention to my diet, trying not to eat sugar, and I avoided sweets altogether. I kept a good exercise regimen, regularly jogging and swimming, and doing some weight lifting.

Therefore, I was in relatively good shape up to the age of forty when I gradually began to experience some health issues here and there, but in the beginning those issues were not significant. I was not paying too much attention to the state of my health and did not consult any doctor to find out was wrong with me. As time went by, my health issues started bothering me more and more. I began having problems with my blood pressure.

It was not that high and, according to modern standards, it was not even supposed to be treated with medication.

Yet it started affecting me, causing unpleasant symptoms like headaches and feeling an unpleasant squeezing sensation all around my head. In the beginning, I was able to control my blood pressure by jogging more frequently, taking a magnesium supplement and trying to meditate from time to time. Meditation was the most difficult part because I was distracted all the time by either external events in my life, or by my own thoughts flooding my consciousness all the time, preventing my attempts to feel more relaxed and content.

Overall, I was able to manage my blood pressure for some time until it became quite high, and I started thinking about going to see a doctor and possibly start taking medication to control it.

In addition, over the months and years, I started experiencing other health issues that were popping up one after another.

I started having bleeding gums, so bad sometimes that I literally could not eat anything. My attempts to clean my teeth brought some

9

relief but only for a while. After several months, they were bleeding again.

I kept going to the dentist to keep cleaning and cleaning, and overall felt very frustrated. I developed some gastrointestinal problems like acid reflux, and felt bloated most of the time. At one point, I felt so bloated that I went to a GI doctor who suggested doing an endoscopy, but I did not like this idea. Instead, I tried fighting this problem by taking health supplements, trying to reorganize my diet, doing yoga exercises, and other things. All those things helped, but only for some time and the bloating and indigestion kept coming back and making me frustrated. In addition, I developed dermatitis.

The most irritating part of it was an itching that was preventing me from sleeping at night and then I felt very tired during the day. I need to mention here that as time went on I started feeling more and more tired.

My energy was somewhat low most of the time and in hindsight I can tell that I felt depressed, irritable and very angry at times.

Overall, I felt quite frustrated and it started affecting my relationships at work and at home.

I knew that something needed to be done about this, but could not focus enough to find a proper solution. In addition to feeling chronically tired and sad, I developed anxiety. I also started gaining some weight, developed chronic insomnia and to my horror, found that I started having problems remembering things. The thought that I was developing some kind of dementia really scared me. To make matters worse, I lost my motivation and ability to experience pleasure in life. Things that were motivating me in the past, like my hobbies, no longer interested me.

I started to see primary care doctors, and different specialists. I was trying to find out what was going wrong with my health and to find proper treatment.

All possible laboratory tests ordered by the doctors were coming back normal and I was given symptomatic treatment for my complaints.

The result was that I ended up with many different pills in my pocket. I took all of them the way they were prescribed. Eventually I started experiencing some side effects. Consequently, I started taking different medications to deal with the side effects caused by the first medications, and soon the number of meds I was taking doubled.

Meanwhile, my health was not improving, even with all these meds. I did get some relief for a short time, but that was it.

I felt sick, frustrated, angry, irritable and helpless about my situation. I felt there had to be a reason why I was experiencing all those symptoms and I needed to find out what that reason was.

My journey to find the answer

I realized that I needed to revive the coping and survival skills I learned while growing up back in the USSR. I now had to use these skills to solve my health issues. At that time I was working a lot, running around, seeing patients and taking care of many other responsibilities.

I made the decision to stop. I arranged for time off.

I isolated myself from all sources of information and communication, things such as TV, cell phone (I told everyone to call me only in case of an emergency), MP3's, tablets, books, magazines and all other sources of information. I walked in the park by the ocean by myself a lot. I did not force myself to think about anything. I was relaxing without being bombarded by information from all over the place all the time, as it used to be. I walked all day long, just coming home to sleep. The reason I did this is that, in the beginning, staying at home and doing nothing was making me feel anxious.

Eventually I got used to it, and in about a week I felt comfortable sitting on the chair in the kitchen or dining room, staring out the window and observing the tree swaying back and forth from the strong wind. I noticed that I started sleeping a little better, but my health overall was not improving and I still experienced the above-mentioned health issues.

The answer: Metabolic Syndrome

One morning I woke up knowing exactly what had been going on with my health. I was in a state of shock because I could not understand why it took me so long to understand this. The answer was a simple one: I was not in touch with myself. I was running around, not able to focus and concentrate. I was distracted by my daily activities. The results of the laboratory tests were all normal — all of this made it impossible to diagnose my health situation.

It became obvious that over those years I had been gradually developing what is known as *Metabolic Syndrome*. *Metabolic Syndrome* has been proven to be one of the main causes of heart attacks and strokes, as well as different types of cancer, and dementia.

What was happening was that my body kept losing its capacity to metabolize carbohydrates. Meanwhile, the pancreas was excreting significant quantities of the hormone insulin, trying to utilize the excess carbs in the bloodstream.

My body was becoming resistant to insulin, and its level in the blood was getting higher and higher. High levels of insulin cause increased inflammation in all tissues and organs. Because of the inflammation, I was experiencing all those above-mentioned symptoms. The pancreas was able to compensate for the excess of carbs in the blood by increasing the amount of insulin excreted, thus the blood sugar levels remained normal. I was not obese. I did not have a high cholesterol level or significantly elevated triglycerides.

I realized why doctors could not understand what was going on with me from a medical scientific point of view: my lab results were normal.

Furthermore, days of measuring fasting insulin blood levels is considered, for some reason, experimental and not practical.

Now that I realized the problem I needed to find a proper solution to heal myself. It was obvious to me that I needed to decrease the amount of the carbohydrates I was consuming daily, but it was not clear yet how to do it.

Finding the healing solution

I went to my favorite park by the ocean and was walking along the shoreline when I remembered the time I had spent time working as a doctor very far north in the USSR. I treated local people who lived off eating only seal meat, fat, and fish, and absolutely nothing else at all. They had a tiny berry that grows for about two weeks a year during springtime and that was it. They were all in very good health, and the most common reason they were seeing me was for different types of traumas they had due to working on the ice.

With that realization, I decided to change my diet. I decided to eat only meat and fish, and nothing else. It was an experiment I chose to conduct on myself without consulting anyone.

However, I want to emphasize repeatedly that **I DO NOT** recommend anyone do anything like I did without consulting a doctor first.

Everyone is unique concerning their genetic make-up, blood type, health issues, religious beliefs, taste preferences and many, many other things.

My book is not about an overall diet. It is about identifying *Metabolic Syndrome* as one of the main causes of different health issues and finding a proper solution to correct the problem. The most appropriate option is to discuss with your primary care doctor the possibility of you having *Metabolic Syndrome* as a cause of your complaints. In addition, it is imperative to consult specialists such as naturopaths, dieticians, and others in the area of alternative medicine in order to be properly diagnosed. It is extremely important NOT TO STOP YOUR MEDICATIONS WITHOUT CONSULTING WITH A DOCTOR FIRST and it is important to be evaluated from different angles by different specialists, and then to follow their recommendations about any diet modification created SPECIFICALLY for you.

What is important to remember is that what is good for me, or what may work for me, may be harmful to you and vice versa. I hope this is well understood at this point by readers.

Therefore, I placed myself on an all meat and fish diet. In the beginning I had some issues with constipation, but it was resolved by chewing food longer and drinking much more water.

Quick improvements and long-term benefits

I noticed a great improvement starting about the beginning of the first week. My blood pressure normalized and has remained normal for the last two years. GI complaints, dermatitis, headaches, bleeding gums – all gone with no trace. My day-to-day energy came back about three to four weeks after I started my new diet and today remains stable at all times. I cannot say that my energy is high, but I cannot say it is low either. It is normal. I no longer experience problems with my memory, and my overall ability to learn and retain new information is working.

I do not feel depressed or anxious anymore. It is normal to react in a certain way to bad and good events in life, but I no longer experience those prolonged low-grade mood episodes tangled-up with anxiety and insomnia.

I started sleeping better by the second week of my new diet and my sleep has remained normal since then.

It has been over two years since I started this new diet. In fact, it is not a diet anymore, it is a new lifestyle I adopted that allows me to feel physically and mentally healthy again. I noticed that I lost the desire to exercise as much as I did before. I do not feel I need as much exercise anymore, and I feel very good just taking a peaceful long walk in the park. It does not mean that I have become weak. I noticed that, on the contrary, I have gained more stamina for long, low intensity exercise, and I lost stamina for high intensity but short exercise.

I eat just once a day, usually at noon or a little later, and the rest of the time I do not feel hungry at all.

I am very mentally active, learning many new things every day and I am happily spending time on my hobbies. I cannot say that my life has become a paradise. I still have my bad days and experience all ranges of emotions. However, I am feeling so much better in all aspects of my life compared to before, adhering to my new diet.

As a psychiatrist, I would like to express my ideas and share my lifetime experience with readers concerning their mental health.

In retrospect

For over twenty-five years, I have seen thousands of patients who were referred to me by primary care providers for psychiatric evaluation and possible treatment. Patients had consulted their primary care providers with physical complaints. Their complaints were diagnosed as psychosomatic. Patients were perceived as anxious, depressed and chronically tired. When I evaluated them, I prescribed medications and followed-up to assess the treatment results.

The term psychosomatic means that a patient has a primary psychiatric problem like, for example, depression and/or anxiety, and complains of physical symptoms that do not have a physical cause, but rather a psychiatric or psychological cause.

At one point in my life, I was advised to see a psychiatrist for the same complaints.

Looking back, I wish I could have talked to my patients about the probable cause of their suffering: *Metabolic Syndrome.*

Many of my patients, however, required psychiatric medications because they had significant mental health issues. However, at the same time, I could have given them some advice as to what they could have done to try to heal themselves. I was not able to do that, simply because I also assumed their problems were psychosomatic in nature.

Today, knowing a lot more and having had my own experience, I talk to some of my patients about the possibility of them having Metabolic Syndrome as one of the probable causes of their mental problems. I also strongly advise them to discuss it with their primary care provider and other specialists, and to follow their recommendations.

Knowledge makes a difference for us in terms of either having a good life or not having a good life and suffering. Having this knowledge is like possessing treasure.

When I remember what I learned in Tibetan hospitals of traditional medicine, I can see now that a change in lifestyle in the right direction, at the right time, can be a lifesaving treatment.

I also remember a specific clinic in the city of Leningrad where I grew up. The doctors in this clinic, internists, psychiatrists and psychologists were treating depression and anxiety disorders by modifying patients' diets, and many patients were recovering quite fast.

Doctors in the clinic were regularly publishing papers in scientific magazines about patients getting better by modifying their diet.

In the olden days, it was a known fact that many illnesses, including mental illness, were caused by excessive consumption of the wrong foods. Knowing that, doctors in the clinic were trying to find the most beneficial diet for each patient. His or her recommendations were unique for each individual.

In the process of treating mental illnesses by modifying the diet, doctors found that many patients stopped complaining about physical symptoms they had been experiencing for years.

Physicians in this clinic were using medications too. It was necessary, taking into account the severity of the mental illnesses patients were suffering from.

However, it was shown in published research papers that many patients were able to successfully decrease the number of psychiatric medications or, in some cases, to stop them altogether and experience a complete remission, due to the modification of their diet.

Depression epidemic: Why?

Depression has reached epidemic proportions these days. Why? It can be explained by the fact that today's lifestyle is very fast; people are burdened by so many different responsibilities, and with constant mental stress from every part of their lives. Too much information bombards our brain, making it work in overdrive. All these things make our lives far more stressful. We must expend huge amounts of mental energy to merely function and keep up with the dynamics of our modern society.

Nevertheless, one of the main factors, and it may be the most important one, that causes depression to reach such an epidemic level is *Metabolic Syndrome*, which I mentioned previously.

Some people are consuming too many carbohydrates that increase insulin levels in the blood.

Recent scientific studies reveal that neurons (brain cells) have insulin receptors designed for the insulin molecule to attach to the cell.

This is needed for the glucose molecule (energy for the cell) to get inside the cell so that it is metabolized as a source of energy for the cell to produce neurotransmitters: the chemicals that allow us to think and experience our world using our sensory faculties.

In response to the increased level of insulin in the bloodstream, the receptors become less sensitive to the insulin molecule and not much glucose can get inside the cell to be used as a source of energy. In addition, there is an enzyme called MAO (a chemical inside the cell) that becomes active because of the impaired glucose metabolism inside the neuron (brain cell).

It quickly destroys a neurotransmitter called dopamine that serves a critical function, particularly for mental health.

The result of developing *Metabolic Syndrome* is a deficiency of the neurotransmitter dopamine. The clinical signs of this deficiency are the following:

1. Lack of energy

2. Lack of motivation

3. Inability to experience pleasure

4. Poor memory, attention and concentration

5. Deficit in problem solving capacity

6. Increase the feeling of wakefulness, insomnia

7. Lack of creativity

8. Feeling bored, sad

It is possible to correct depression with the help of specific antidepressant medications, and it needs to be done. However, Metabolic Syndrome, if not corrected, will further worsen depression and then the dosage of depression medication needs to be corrected appropriately.

At some point in time a patient might even stop responding to the antidepressant and require either a change of medication, or to add another or several other medications to be able to control the signs of depression.

Furthermore, if the main problem *(Metabolic Syndrome)* is still not addressed, then it is possible that the patient may stop responding to the medications completely and would then require a different type of treatment, like Electro-convulsive therapy.

Metabolic Syndrome also disrupts the synthesis of the other neurotransmitters that are important for mental health. Some of these vital neurotransmitters are serotonin, norepinephrine, acetylcholine, and many others. The lack of these chemicals in the brain will eventually lead to depression.

Using your intuition

You can talk to specialists about traditional and alternative medicine, and get all sorts of opinions about making changes in your lifestyle (diet, exercise, and other changes) in order to regain your health. However, the ultimate consultant is you. It really does not matter if you have no special knowledge in these health related areas. What you do have is intuition and it is needed, in addition to all the information from consultations. Your intuition will tell you the right thing to do for yourself. Unfortunately, intuition is greatly suppressed by the information noise that surrounds us everywhere we go. And more frequently than not, we create a noise level ourselves in an attempt to escape from thinking about different issues and problems in our everyday life. It would be an excellent idea to try to do everything possible to decrease this noise and try to listen to a higher aspect of yourself – intuition.

I remember the time I traveled to Tibet with a group of doctors. The purpose was to get to know the local culture and attend lectures about Tibetan traditional herbal medicine.

I asked one of the doctors to describe to me what usually happens when a patient walks into his office for an evaluation.

The doctor explained that he and the patient sit next to each other for at least five minutes, meditating. He explained that this is mandatory and helps with communication, as they get further into the session. He made it clear that meditation is needed for the patient to calm down and to get emotions and thoughts in check to be able to clearly explain what seems to be the problem. He said that, based on his experience, it is much easier to accurately diagnose a patient after a meditation session. He added that his meditation helps him *feel out the patient* better.

When I asked him what that means, he explained that he usually starts feeling intuitively and can feel what is wrong with the patient and what organ of the body needs attention, at that particular moment.

So why is your intuition important? Because it allows you to be aware of your state of health and overall wellbeing. Intuition will connect you to the higher aspect of yourself, to the source of all knowledge.

People spend their life rushing from one activity to another, grabbing at things, trying to achieve what is sometimes impossible.

Meanwhile, they are not able to listen to their intuition which has probably been trying to tell them it is time to stop rushing, and that if they do not stop, some sort of disaster will most likely strike very soon.

What about meditation?

I would like to talk about meditation and explain why it is important to practice it daily, from a mental health point of view.

In this book, I do not want to replicate the many pages that have already been written about meditation and the different techniques. You can easily spend the rest of your life just reading about this subject.

However, I do want to mention the recent research findings about meditation and mental health.

Research demonstrates that people who have meditated for a long time (over a year) are able to produce up to sixty percent more of the dopamine neurotransmitter in comparison with people who started meditation only recently. I have discussed the important role of dopamine, so you can draw your own conclusion. People who have been meditating for a long time say that it makes them feel happier, and now you can understand why this is.

At this point, I would like to mention several things about meditation. I have been meditating for a long time and over the years, I have been seeing and talking to different people (my patients and others, like my friends) who have been meditating for some time or gave up meditation for some reason, and I came to some conclusions regarding meditation.

First, I would like to mention that meditation can be hard work. If someone thinks it is just about relaxing, this is far from the truth. You have to use certain techniques to be able to reach a state of mind where you experience no thoughts at all, or just rare random thoughts you easily can push away. It can be very hard and sometimes a person needs to use a specific method of meditation (for example, repeating a mantra or concentrating on breathing) for a long, long, time before being able to reach a calm and thoughtless state of mind.

Usually a big fight happens between trying to reach a state of calm and the person's own thoughts that try to prevent him/her from being able to concentrate on the objective of the meditation.

To overcome this challenge, you need to develop an understanding of meditation, have willpower, and a lot of patience. However, the reward is tremendous.

In addition, after meditating for some time, you might start to experience negative emotions like anger and irritability, and even start feeling sad and anxious. This is normal. It means that all those negative emotions are trying to leave your body and mind. During these periods, it is helpful to increase the amount of exercise in your daily routine – it will speed up the healing process.

It is important to meditate every day. Meditation is like taking medication. It works best if you do it every day and preferably at the same time each day.

To maximize the effect of your meditation, it is best to create a special place in your house designated for your meditation time. Consider it a sacred place. You can decorate this place with anything you like.

Practice shows that a person usually reaches a meditative state of mind much faster and the quality of meditation is much deeper if it happens in your personally created sanctuary.

If you are in good mental health, daily meditation is an excellent therapeutic tool. It will ensure you will not relapse into mental illness if or when affected by stress. It is important to state that if a person is able to design a diet that helps him/her to get rid of *Metabolic Syndrome* that person should, in addition to this, be able to meditate on a regular basis. This creates a path to overall good health, based on my personal experience.

CHAPTER 3

Stages of recovery

You will go through several stages on the path to recovery:

Stage 1

First, you have to notice that something is wrong with your health. You then need to pay attention to the signs, or symptoms of the illness. Surprisingly, most people are so engaged in their daily activities and responsibilities that they miss the signs completely or do not pay attention to them, thinking that nothing serious is going on.

Stage 2

You need to acknowledge the fact that you have some health issues that need to be addressed. For some reason, many people exist in a state of complete denial of this problem.

In this case, one needs to do some deep psychological work to sort things out and find answers as to why.

Stage 3

You need to take responsibility for your health and recovery. This means you need to do everything possible, including consulting with every possible specialist to find out what is going on with your health. You need to discuss with your primary care provider and other specialists the possibility that you are developing or have Metabolic Syndrome, as one of the explanations for the symptoms.

Stage 4

Try to consult with every possible specialist in order to design a specific diet for your lifestyle that will keep your symptoms in check.

Stage 5

Incorporate daily meditation into your life.

What is the other most important cause of Metabolic Syndrome besides the increased consumption of carbs? It is obvious: chronic mental and emotional poisoning fueled by the excess of information coming from mass media.

In that regard there is no difference between being poisoned with drugs or by information. In both cases, you experience tremendous physical and mental stress. Stress causes your stress hormones to shoot up which in turn causes blood glucose levels to increase, which in turn elevates insulin levels. As I mentioned before, the chronically elevated insulin levels produce changes in your body that lead to the development of all sorts of modern-age diseases.

Surprisingly again, most people do not perceive information poisoning as a stress factor. Actually, the addiction to modern technology seems to make people feel good. What they do not understand is that they are stressing themselves by, for example, having their cell phone next to them twenty-four hours a day.

My strong advice to these people is to gradually start removing themselves from that type of stress. By doing this, they will greatly diminish the chances of developing *Metabolic Syndrome.*

Most of the time this cannot be done immediately. People who are addicted to drugs, for example, have to withdraw gradually in order to avoid intense withdrawal symptoms. Depending on the substance, it sometimes can only be done in a clinical setting while being closely monitored by doctors to prevent possible life threatening withdrawal symptoms. The same withdrawal concept applies to being addicted to information. Information is a material substance and can be manipulated, sent, stored, and changed, as any other material substance in this world. It is not something abstract, it is very much concrete.

I recommend to initially start to withdraw from your cell phone. I know, based on my personal experience, that this can be very difficult and turn into an anxiety-provoking thing to do, so it has to be done slowly.

I suggest you start by not carrying it with you for part of the day. For example, when you are at work and, in case of an emergency, someone can contact you by calling your work phone extension.

Do it for a week or two until you feel comfortable, not restless, and it does not create too much anxiety. Then, later, you may choose to not carry your phone whenever you go outside your home. As an example, do some shopping or take a walk by yourself or with someone else without your phone. Do it for two to three weeks, and at the end of the first month you will see and feel that you have become calmer, and more content. It will help if you also take nature walks. Nature's positive energy will lift your spirit and speed up the healing process of your withdrawal symptoms from information poisoning.

When you start feeling better, you can design your own program of how to withdraw from the rest of mass media such as TV, radio, tablets and other devices. You need to commit to using all these electronic devices strictly for business purposes, and nothing else.

In the process of doing this, you will see that not only have you calmed down emotionally, but, by getting in touch with the higher aspect of yourself, you are becoming more intuitive.

You become more intuitive which means that you know what to do and how to react to situations in your life. Your creative mind wakes up and generates more valuable ideas to implement in your everyday life and future projects.

To withdraw from mass media is the most powerful meditation technique you can use.

Leonid Altshuler

Withdrawal symptoms: How to deal with anxiety and restlessness

Increase the amount of physical activity, drink plenty of water, do not eat many sweets, talk to people who are next to you, like family members, and take nature walks.

Metabolic Syndrome: why so many cases?

Many cases can most likely be attributed to psychological reasons such as anxiety. The constant worry about what is going to happen in life, from worry about the property people possess, to the car they have, and the bank account if they get sick. People try to surround themselves with all possible insurance policies, but still worry constantly because they have to pay for all these insurance policies. Who will pay if they get sick? Compounding these issues are the children who need money for education. What will happen to the children if you run out of money to give to them?

I am not saying anything good or bad about countries that have socialized medicine and a free education system. Every system has pluses and minuses. However, I can say that constant worry (the worry may not be even at a conscious level)

36

causes chronic stress, and the result of this type of situation has been discussed.

I do not make any recommendation as to how it is possible to avoid such stress, but I think daily meditation, when it is done correctly, can decrease anxiety levels no matter what caused the anxiety in the first place. Practicing meditation will make you feel happier whether your life situation is bad or good.

Feeling disconnected from others can be another cause of chronic stress. This situation is often created because of the overuse of electronic equipment. Whether they realize it or not, people start missing one-on-one human relationships. It is imperative for good mental health to be engaged in non-electronic relationships. Humans involuntarily rely on each other to protect themselves from the hazards of the environment they live in. Humans evolved this way millions of years ago, and nothing has changed since then.

When your only relationship is with your cell phone and computer, you are prone to feeling insecure, alone, anxious, even scared. It even causes feelings of sadness.

The latest research data shows that people who spend most of their time on websites such as social media websites are sadder and more anxious compared with other people who do not. Those who spend more time on the internet increase their level of stress in their daily lives.

Therefore, the point is for you to be able to engage in normal, non-electronic relationships with other humans as much as possible. You can do this maybe by attending more meet-up groups, depending on your individual situation, hobbies and interests. Participating in these human activities will decrease the level of stress you have been chronically experiencing, even though you might not be aware of it.

Generosity and (self) compassion

In many cultures, giving up something to someone else who needs it more than us, or generosity to others, has long been considered a "good act" or "good deed", part of our responsibility as civilized and evolved beings. Today in our society this gesture is often forgotten as our fast lifestyle often bypasses simple acts of compassion and giving. Perhaps it is time to revisit this concept and start at home, in ourselves. For example, giving up food, or fasting (consult your doctor before doing it) one day a week, or donating money to different religious and non-religious institutions of your choice, may contribute to a holistic feeling of well-being. Our ancestors, for thousands or more years, believed in God and prayed to God on a daily basis. I think we have in our DNA the desire to believe in a higher power, and to pray.

I also think it is imperative for good mental health to continue praying to a God (whoever you believe in, based on your religious preference). I believe that not doing so causes us to feel more anxious.

However, this is just my hypothesis.

CHAPTER 4

The value of focus and clarity

Some can write a book of 1,000 pages and say nothing at all. Very often, this is what actually happens. Brevity is the soul of wit. However, a book has to sell, which is why it should be heavy and contain many pages. That way the reader spends hours, days, months and years trying to clarify the meaning buried under heaps of needless information that can be easily found anywhere on the Internet and elsewhere. Even if these books discuss the most recent scientific information, it will only beat the reader down by the sheer volume of information and will not give him/her a chance to focus on the main issue.

The essence of a book should be practical recommendations that can be IMPLEMENTED. A book should be written without excessive verbal garbage.

Why am I saying this?

Because in this book you will find the essence. Yes, it has just a few pages and you can hardly call it a full-fledged book. However, it contains something that will be of value to you: the essence and the basics without any surplus information.

Prelude to meditation

One challenging reality of modern life is the rapid speed of life. To mentally and physically keep yourself distracted from the direct and spontaneous daily routines and problems can be hard. To do this, you need to involve two human components: the external and the internal environments. The external one is quite clear. The inner one includes different qualities of your nature like willingness, persistence, willpower etc. Can many people say that life circumstances are always in favor of them? I guess not.

That is exactly why most people are initially enthusiastic about yoga, meditation and practicing different Eastern methods but eventually, they leave it behind or do not do it regularly and that does not lead to success.

The high speed of life makes it hard to concentrate and to find time and energy. This is undisputed.

Suggested meditation techniques

Do you identify with any or all of these questions and statements?

Why am I not calm and happy?

Why am I always worried about the future?

Why is the past bothering me so much?

I cannot enjoy life; I am in a constant rush.

I am tired of chaos and the meaningless of everything that is going on.

The goals I reach do not give me the desired satisfaction.

I am always searching for something else and I am unsatisfied.

I need something bigger, newer, and more expensive.

I cannot relax.

I am afraid to lag behind in this rat race. I fear I will be left by the roadside.

I do not sleep well.

My mood is low.

I am always annoyed, I am not pleased and I can even be aggressive.

As time goes by, these problems seem to get worse.

Sometimes I want to give up everything and leave the village. Nevertheless, I cannot.

Lastly...

What should I do? I do not want to take medication. No! Psychiatric medications are not for me. I have tried it once. I was sick all the time ... Doctor, please give me any advice, please help me...

If you can identify with any of these statements and questions, this meditation technique will be of help to you. One advantage of my method is that you do not need to create a specific time and place to do the exercise. It fits in perfectly with the lifestyle of any modern civilized human being.

What is the goal of the method?

To reach and live in a constant calm and happy condition.

Is this goal achievable? Yes, of course

I am telling you this as an expert in psychiatry who has treated thousands of patients for twenty-five years.

Do not worry, you will find nothing about medication or psychotherapy in this book. I am not going to talk about the recent achievements of psychiatry and related sciences. In addition, I will not touch upon anything metaphysical, astral or mystic. I pursue a different objective.

You should learn a few undeniable truths. The practice suggests that any information is much easier to sink in if it is repeated several times. In this case, it is easier to learn it and remember it.

What is the purpose of this method?

I want to offer you a special method that will let you become calm, satisfied and happy for a short time.

Note, however, that the constant practical application of this method will result in the above-mentioned emotional state to become continuous and constant. As you practice this method over time, it will start working for you, regardless of whether you practice it consciously or not. This is important to understand.

Let me repeat: At a certain stage of doing the exercises, the method will become the triggering mechanism for your state of good mood even without conscious implementation. Here the principle of a conditioned reflex will work. I will explain it in more detail later.

Important points to keep in mind

Now I would like to focus on a few points that the reader should pay close attention to, read a few times and try to understand completely.

1. All emotional disorders originate from biological reasons. They have an underlying

cause. Hepatitis implies liver problems. Pyelonephritis – kidney problems.
Depression means that the root of the problem is in the brain.

2. Emotional problems come from the inefficient functioning of neurotransmitters in the brain and the shortage or abundance of them, as well as their incorrect cooperation and the invalid functioning of the nerve cell receptors in the brain.
I repeat that they come from biological reasons. The external world situations are only a triggering mechanism that starts the process that reveals itself as a disease.

3. Besides dopamine, one of the basic neurotransmitters defining our mood is serotonin.

4. Serotonin is produced and accumulated in nerve cells mostly at night or in the daytime when you close your eyes or when you meditate. When you are awake, serotonin is consumed. The more stressful your life is, the faster it is consumed and the slower it is produced and accumulated.

The shortage of serotonin is linked with the state of depression.

5. Our brain works in different rhythms.
Serotonin is synthesized and accumulated mostly in the Alpha rhythm of our brain.
You might have noticed that children, especially young toddlers up to twelve years old are usually happy, unless adults or other children bully them.
This is explained by the fact that the brain at this age is mostly working in Alpha. Interestingly, most children ten to twelve years old do not think in abstract categories (like past and future events); they live only in the present, right here, right now. Alpha brainwaves are interconnected with attention to what is going on here and now. Therefore, when you concentrate on current events you trigger Alpha brainwaves.

6. Meditation generates Alpha brainwaves. In this state, a human being subjectively feels inner calmness and absence of any other thoughts.

CHAPTER 5

The Altshuler Method

Every day we perform actions that are necessary for us to live our life. These actions are performed automatically without thinking, every day during our entire life. For example, waking up in the morning, getting up from bed, walking around in our apartment, cleaning teeth, shaving, taking a shower, drying our body with a towel, eating, drinking, getting dressed. These actions are the foundation of the method.

Implementation of the method

The method is practiced over time because you will have to adjust to your new life in the full meaning of the words, and to the unfamiliar perception of your newly perceived environment. Your conscious mind will therefore need time to adjust to these changes.

First Week

In the morning. You wake up. You go to the bathroom. Make sure that all your attention is focused on the sense you have when the toothbrush is touching your teeth and gums. It is important to keep your conscious attention during the entire process of cleaning your teeth. If something distracts you, gently pull your attention back to cleaning teeth. You should also focus your attention on rinsing your mouth after the teeth cleaning. Men can apply this focusing exercise on shaving.

The whole process can take one or two minutes, but for your brain it is enough to start changes into the Alpha brainwaves.

Do this task or exercise for the first week. Do not do anything else.

Second Week

Every morning, continue focusing on cleaning your teeth and rinsing your mouth. Starting this second week, let us add focusing on taking a shower. Hold your attention to the sensations you have when the water touches your body. Try to sustain this attention to the water touching your body during the entire time you take a shower. When you are done, dry yourself with a towel. All your attention should be focused on your body sensations when the towel dries it. As I said in the beginning, if you notice your attention switching to something else slowly focus it back on the towel drying your skin. Do not get upset if it is difficult to do. Each time you repeat the exercise it will become easier.

Third Week

During this third week, continue to do what you did every morning for the first two weeks. In addition, this week, you will start to concentrate on eating and drinking. Start with breakfast. You should concentrate on the taste sensations and the process of chewing the food.

However, again, do not get upset if your attention starts to slip away. Just get it back in focus.

Fourth Week

This fourth week, continue to do what you have been doing every morning for the first three weeks, but also start to focus on walking around your living area. Focus on the sensations you have when touching the floor with both feet. Try to focus your attention on your feet.

Try this at least for the first half hour as soon as you get up.

Therefore, after a month you will have these four exercises to do every morning. You will see and feel the changes you are going through in your mind. These changes are related to your emotional background and the process of perception of everything that we call reality in our everyday life.

Your morning Alpha brainwaves will enhance your entire day by feeling good and calm.

At a certain stage, you will get feedback. This is an important point it is necessary to understand.

Walking, washing, eating, will have become the triggering mechanism that will automatically switch your brain into Alpha.

In other words, you will not have to constantly concentrate on the sensations coming from these four actions to make your brain work in Alpha. It will happen by itself, automatically, when you start eating, walking, cleaning your teeth or taking a shower.

However, it is important to know that if you do not sustain this condition of being conscious of your walking, eating, etc. for a long period the effect tends to disappear gradually. Therefore, I recommend that you practice some of these specific exercises from time to time. You can continue doing all four of them or only three or two, or just do the one you like the most. In addition, you can practice them not only in the morning but also in the afternoon or in the evening, for example, when you are walking in the street.

Positive changes to expect

Now I am going to share with you the positive changes that I saw in my patients.

Emotional Stress

First, the state of emotional stress disappears. Patients gain a feeling of serenity. Troubles seem to go away. Finally, the depression goes away too. They gain a feeling of optimism and their creativity improves. Concentration and memory both improve.

Individuals feel they have more energy than before. Their relationships at work and at home improve. They sleep better. All the above-mentioned results come from the increase and dominance of Alpha waves in your brain.

I believe this is the best possible method that is adjusted for our modern crazy speed of life. This method offers people a relatively simple and quick escape from their emotional crisis. More importantly, it also provides them with a tool that can keep at bay possible states of neurosis.

An alternative scenario

For those who can find time and a place to exercise by themselves, here is another method. It does not mean that these people cannot practice what I described in the first part; it is just an additional opportunity, another way to go.

In this method, the actual time and place are the most important healing factors. Let me explain what I mean. Modern life and its hectic rhythm gives a person enormous emotional and physical stress.

Actually, it is not correct to separate these two levels, because if you look deeper, the physical and the emotional parts are one. Let us try to separate them. Stress causes both emotional and physical inhibitions. Emotional ones are accumulated in the subconscious, and the physical ones show up as muscle stress. Your body tries to keep the energies balanced so it is trying to get rid of negativity.

However, to do that, negativity needs to make its way to the conscious. In other words, for the negative emotions to leave your body, they have to come to the surface, to the conscious, from the level of the subconscious, and actually be experienced.

Of course, this can come with painful psychological experiences. In the same way, your body is trying to get rid of muscle stress by sending you signals as pain sensations here and there. Unfortunately, we often ignore them, and do not pay attention.

When the unconscious throws out another serving of negativity into the conscious, the person feels that negativity. It can manifest in different ways: nervousness, fear, despair, or anger.

In response to that, the person usually shifts his or her attention to anything else around to be distracted from the negativity. The distraction can be anything, such as another person, an animal or any other creature or object. Most often computers, phones and TVs attract our attention.

This shift from the conscious gives your body an opportunity to bury the negativity again into the unconscious, thus creating a state of avoidance so that you do not experience the negativity. This process is an infinite one that happens many times a day.

This is why so many people are not able to communicate with themselves. They need to shift to something else all the time, and it has to be something from the external environment. That is how a person ends up fighting with him/herself. However, perhaps surprisingly, eventually the negativity wins, because it starts to affect the endocrine and the immune systems, causing diseases that sometimes are lethal.

The question is what to do?

The answer is, do NOTHING. Literally nothing.

Now I am going to tell you how to do nothing because it can be very difficult, but at the same time, it could not be simpler.

Description of alternative method

It is important to choose a time when you are at home alone or nobody can disturb you.

Choose a room. Lay something soft on the floor near the wall to make it comfortable for sitting and lying. Now remove all the electronic devices from the room including TV and radio, all the newspapers, and magazines. The most important thing is that you remove everything that can distract you, everything that can draw your attention. Sit down near the wall and make yourself comfortable. You should sit with your back to the window. Therefore, you are sitting down. Note that you do not need to focus on anything. There is a familiar room in front of you; you have seen it a thousand times. Maybe there is a bed across from you, maybe it is a bookcase or a table.

You can think about anything you like. You can change your position as many times as you like. You may even lie down.

The most important condition is to not move from the place, and do not do any exercise.

Just be there. If you are tired of sitting like this, change the pose. Change it as many times as you want. Look wherever you want. If you feel sleepy, lie down and sleep. When you wake up continue sitting there.

This exercise requires staying in the same place you have chosen, for thirty minutes a day.

Thirty minutes will give the best results. If you cannot do thirty, do at least twenty minutes, which is the minimum. Do this any time of day. Of course, it is better not to do it too late at night because you will feel sleepy.

Explanation

The purpose of this exercise is to stay in one place while there is no opportunity to distract you and thus push the negativity back inside. Eventually you will realize and experience unpleasant emotions. It can be anything - nervousness, anger, sadness, depression, etc. It is important to give yourself a chance to experience these. Once you do, these emotions will go away. If you feel overcome with anger, you should take a pillow and beat it as hard as you want. If you feel depressed, be with it; let yourself cry, if you want. If you suddenly want to laugh, you should laugh as much as you want. Try to be ready for any demonstration of emotions that emerge from inside your mind.

Sometimes you will be overcome with the desire to stand up and do something immediately. Fight it, do not let the negativity win.

You can change your position as often as you want. The most important thing is to feel comfortable.

If you want to be there in one place more than twenty minutes, stay there as long as you want.

The best way to do this exercise is every day at the same time. Every day. Do it for at least a month. I can assure you that at a certain stage of the exercise you will feel a strong emotional relief. You should continue because you will eventually reach a point when you feel all thoughts have disappeared and you are very calm. It is a signal that you (your brainwaves) are in Alpha. This is the state where one of the most important chemical molecules, serotonin, is synthesized and accumulated. Serotonin generates a good mood, optimism, and energy. The more you practice the faster you will reach this Alpha-rhythm.

Can this method be called meditation?

To some extent, yes. Nevertheless, with my exercise you do not have to learn anything new. You do not have to learn how to stay in one position, or even how to focus on breathing etc.

I am certain that for a modern human being, especially for the ones who live in a big industrial city, the usual kind of meditation is highly undesirable.

The reason is that concentrating on anything (in this case on oneself) will only push the negativity deeper inside. Normal meditations are good for people who live, for example, in the mountains of Tibet in relatively calm and non-stressful conditions.

On the other hand, if practicing my method results in calmness and stress resistance for you, then you can try other methods of meditation if you want.

So, now you have a method for doing nothing.

A few words about rushing

What prevents us from living in harmony with everything? What deprives us of the opportunity to see beautiful things around us? The answer is rush.

Human beings are eager to be on time. We have big demands, we consume big quantities, we go big distances, and we get big headaches.

Is there a way to slow down?

Of course there is.

Autohypnosis

Autohypnosis, or verbal formulas, are methods that have been tested many times and it undoubtedly works.

Autohypnosis works best when you do it before going to bed and in the morning when you wake up. Verbal formulas should be spoken, three times each. The main thing is to pronounce them very slowly. What is even more important is feel deeply the state you want to achieve. For example, if you say aloud the phrase "I AM ALWAYS COMPLETELY RELAXED", you should arouse the feeling of relaxation in your body while you are saying the words.

Here are those verbal formulas necessary to reprogram your brain not to rush. I repeat, you should say them very slowly and three times in a row:

I AM NEVER IN A RUSH FOR ANYTHING. I AM NEVER
IN A HURRY TO ANYWHERE.

I AM DOING EVERYTHING SLOWLY, SLOWLY, SLOWLY.

I AM ALWAYS RELAXED IN MY MIND.

Say these words at least twice a day, before going to bed and after you wake up, and you will see very quickly that you will become much calmer and, most surprisingly, that you have time to do many more things than before without getting very tired.

Again, most of the time it is related to the gradual shift of your brain functioning in Alpha.

You should understand that if you change one thing in your life you automatically change everything. In this case, you will see positive changes at all levels.

This is because you are on the right path, you are on the way to rest, relaxation and contemplation — and all these aspects are essential for productivity, creativity and success.

Otherwise, what is the point of being successful if you are stressed and not able to enjoy your life because you always rush somewhere?

The most important thing you can do for your health

Sometimes I wonder: What would be one of the most important things one could do for their health issues?

I know the answer. You need to meditate. Meditation is a concept much broader than what is written in most books, and it is important that you understand this.

Why breaking routines is healthy

Meditation is any process or activity that breaks a routine behavior pattern. A routine, or a specific pattern of behavior that is repeated day after day, month after month, year after year, brings a sense of security. It is predictable, and therefore nothing unexpected happens, no danger, life goes on uninterrupted. It means that your body does not need to go into survival mode. What is the survival mode in charge of? It is responsible for heightened senses, increased attention and concentration. It is also involved in the process of finding creative solutions when circumstances suddenly change. Dopamine is one of several neurotransmitters responsible for the process of this adaptation to a new situation.

Any change in a routine creates a sense of insecurity. You may not even be aware of it.

In order to navigate to the safety of an exit, to escape from a potentially dangerous situation, or to help you adjust to a new environment, your brain will start producing more dopamine. As a result, both your attention and concentration increase, which means you become more alert and kick-start the creative process of problem solving.

You already know the benefits of increased levels of dopamine in the brain.

How to break routine

One way to keep dopamine levels high is to start a new meditation technique that breaks the pattern of a routine. It does not have to be anything extraordinary, like traveling to Mt. Everest or anything like that. It can be much simpler. For example, try to get home from work by taking a new route. Try to wake up in the morning thirty minutes earlier and spend the extra time any way you like. Create and add to your daily routine one new thing every day. You will like some of the changes you make and will not like some of the others. You will probably like to keep doing something you like, but at the same time, try to find another activity that interests you.

This also applies to intellectual activities and pursuits. For example, let us say you want to learn about Napoleon. Start by reading articles about him. Then the next day you can continue reading about Napoleon.

A new subject may fascinate you and switch your attention to something else like reading about gardening, or dogs and cats, or anything else that might potentially interest you.

The result is that your life will no longer be boring, and the increased level of dopamine will force you to discover new things in life until, at some point, you will be completely engaged in a creative process.

I am not saying that you need to change things every day, but you need to find new avenues for your development, both physical and intellectual. Try to break a routine whenever you can and wherever you can, so that your dopamine levels stay in the healthy and HAPPY range.

Why do you feel better emotionally when you are on a vacation? Because you break routines.

Anything that breaks a routine and creates a healthy level of insecurity is good for your mental and physical health. Making new discoveries every day is an excellent way of keeping yourself happy and motivated.

Cave dwellers did not have issues with routines because they had to keep making changes every day to fight for survival in their harsh and dangerous environment.

Our bodies are programmed to function at a normal level only when they are under low-grade stress, like continuously having to adapt to a constantly changing environment.

Why is meditation so important?

You may wonder why I consider meditation such an important activity compared with anything else.

Daily meditation, done properly in the early morning, presets your thinking pattern and, consequently, the pattern of all your actions for the rest of the day.

When you wake up and rush to start your day, you usually have some idea as to which things are of importance. Most importantly, you have some priority system in your mind about the importance of all your activities planned for the day. For example, you probably consider going to work as the number one thing that needs to be done. Then, spending time with your children in the evening is the thing that has number two on your priority scale.

Number three might be to walk the dog. Number four could be watching a program on TV. The next item down your priority list might be to read a book, and it can go on, and on, until the last thing to do might be to call your old friend.

Long-term effects of meditation

What happens after you have been meditating for some time every morning? You will see that things you had planned to do in a specific sequence during the day are completely changed concerning their order of importance.

For example, you may find that taking a walk in the park after you get home from work might become the number one priority. Then, reading an article about Buddhism and the meaning of life might become number two priority. Calling your friend jumps up to number three.

You may even realize that the most important thing for you to do is to consider changing your job because you do not feel it is rewarding anymore.

Meditation creates a direct contact with your TRUE needs so you can live in harmony with yourself and with the environment around you.

About prioritizing

Modern life detaches people from themselves and forces them to run around trying to accomplish things that are expected of them. However, frequently, those things are not the ones that are good for someone who is mentally and physically healthy.

The task is to find out what is the most important, number one thing for you to do, and make sure you do it first, while making proper adjustments so that you are still functioning within modern society. This is not a simple task, but, at least, through this process you become more clearly aware of your personal values and needs.

This knowledge will also help create a new healthy lifestyle that will not only benefit you, but also the people who live with you.

The only way to live a harmonious life is to take meditation seriously and do it every day. Meditation must become your number ONE priority each day.

As you may have noticed, I do not get tired of repeating the same thing constantly! If your purpose is to feel content with your life (happiness is an extreme emotion, and rarely can someone be happy all the time) then you need to focus your attention on meditation.

Why is it difficult for me to commit to daily meditation?

I want to explain here why it is very difficult for so many people to commit themselves to a meditation routine.

It is because we live in an environment where people and things move extremely fast. Every person lives off their natural survival instincts, which humans acquired millions of years ago.

This instinct tells us that we, in order to able to survive, need to adjust to the environment we live in.

It means that we need to adjust our speed to everyone else's speed, otherwise, if we slow down, we will be left behind without the support of the crowd and anything could then happen to us. Our survival instinct does not care that we live in a civilized society, surrounded by plenty of food and with places where we can hide from the cold or heat, or any other natural hazard.

Our survival instinct sees us as a life form left behind by our own species, and therefore we need to protect ourselves from environmental dangers that could kill us.

When we slow down our life speed by meditation, we usually start to experience some uncomfortable emotions, and very quickly we have the urge to keep moving, speeding, trying to catch up with the crowd.

Understanding that these urges and emotions are part of the process will reassure you and allow you to continue your meditation program and to be successful with it.

As a psychiatrist, I know that it is purely good luck to be born with genes that resist life stress, which would mean you have a nice life and do not experience significant problems with depression and anxiety. Unfortunately, not many people are that lucky. The only way to develop a resistance to stress and decrease your chances of developing some type of mental illness is to practice meditation on a daily basis.

You have to practice it whether you are in a bad mood or a good mood.

My experience tells me that people who meditate regularly are less prone to developing a relapse of a mental illness.

The way to feeling content: change your lifestyle

The mental state does not exist separately from the physical. They both represent ONE thing.

Feeling content and healthy is a big reward that comes with hard work, unless you are born with "happy genes".

Personally, I decided to make a change in my life. Yes, it was a big challenge in the beginning.

I am now rewarded by being free of suffering what was making me feel miserable for so long.

This book is not about how to become healthier by incorporating and following a new diet, or how to become happier by meditating daily, or about following any other program to improve one's life. This book is about you searching for a new lifestyle. It is about starting a new way of life that is comfortable for you at all levels.

How do I find a diet that is right for me?

Let us discuss the issue of diet. Let us imagine that you need a pair of shoes because your old ones are worn out. You search for shoes that meet your personal criteria. They have to be of a suitable size, relatively light, a color that you like, made of the material that you like, and be comfortable because you plan to wear those shoes as long as you can. The same applies to diet. There are four main criteria, in my opinion, that are important to consider when figuring out what is the proper way for you to eat:

> 1. You need to eat as much as you want, and not feel hungry soon after. In this case, your insulin level is steady and does not bring down your blood sugar level, and as a result, you do not experience hunger. You will not gain any weight, simply because, since you do not feel hungry, you will not eat as frequently.
> 2. You do not miss the food you used to like. You do not think about it, dream about it or talk about it.

3. Your overall energy level is steady. It does not fly up and down throughout the day and you do not feel tired and sleepy.

4. You do not become obsessed with constantly counting calories and percentages of proteins, fats, and carbs in your diet, and start living with a calculator in your pocket. That kind of life in itself would be stressful for anyone.

If you have all these four components taken care of, then you can say that you have developed a new lifestyle you can adhere to indefinitely.

If you start dieting, and for one reason or another it makes you uncomfortable, it means that your current diet or new way of eating needs to be modified, or even completely changed. Try another diet recommended for you based on your unique individual needs. Keep trying different diets until you find the right one for you.

The same applies to meditation. You may try hundreds of different techniques and then find that nothing suits you. You may get so tired and frustrated after trying out so many different methods and techniques that you start thinking about giving up, but do not give up.

Eventually you will find that unique technique that is a good fit with who you are and what you like to do.

This concept applies to everything in life, including searching for a life partner. Just keep looking. Do not compromise on things that do not make you feel good or comfortable.

Closing words

Finding a lifestyle that is healthy for you is the path to feeling content. Not happy, not sad, but content, and that is what humanity has been trying to find for millennia – contentment. But it is so difficult!

Have you ever wondered why it is so difficult for people to find a lifestyle that suits their unique personalities?

It is because we do not hear the voice of intuition that keeps trying to tell us about the most important things we should do to feel content. Why do we not hear this little voice? Because of the white noise caused by the information that blasts us every second of our life from every direction. Therefore, what we need to do is to eliminate all this noise so we can hear the voice of our intuition again.

You need to stop running around trying to catch something or find somebody to make you feel good.

I did stop. Moreover, when I stopped I found what I was looking for, for so many years. I firmly believe that if I can do it, then anyone can do it.

The most important thing is – you need to be motivated. I hope very much that my tiny book has helped you to feel this way.

Leonid Altshuler, M.D.

www.ingramcontent.com/pod-product-compliance
Lightning Source LLC
Chambersburg PA
CBHW070911280326
41934CB00008B/1678